I0412123

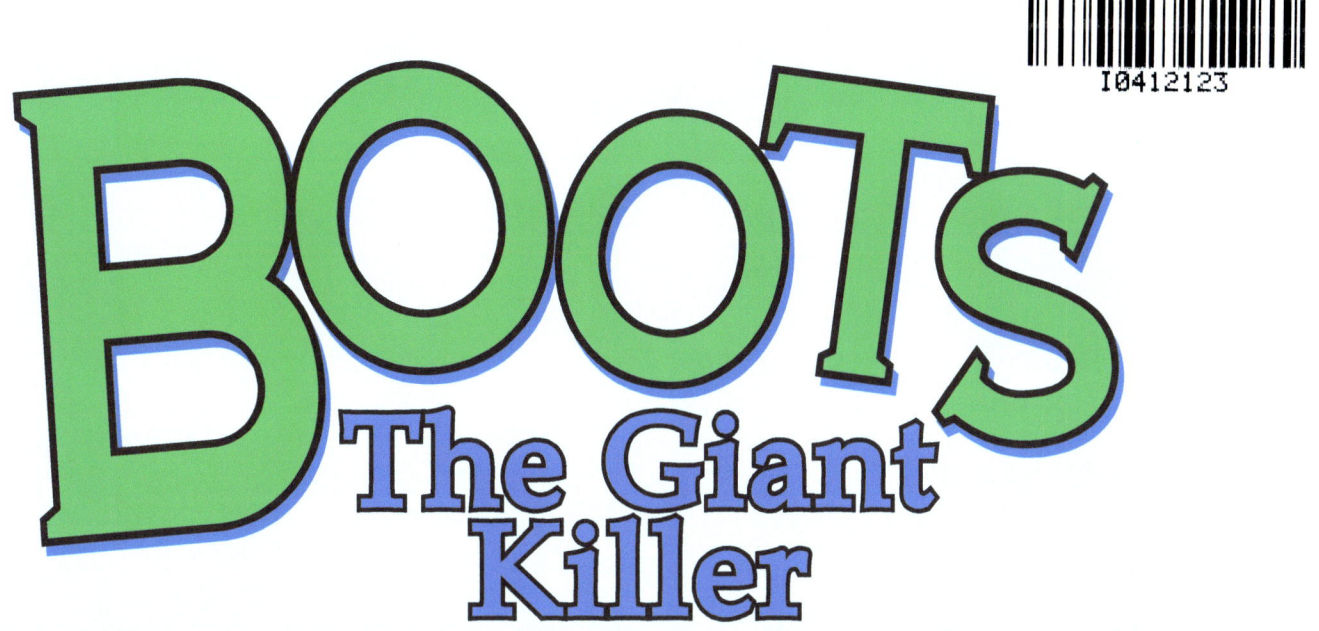

BOOTs The Giant Killer

An Upbeat Analogy About Diabetes

Book Three of the You Can Do It! Series

Written by   Eleanor Troutt
Illustrated by   Rob Peters

BOOTS THE GIANT KILLER
An Upbeat Analogy About Diabetes

Written by Eleanor Troutt
Illustrated by Rob Peters

This is the third book in the YOU CAN DO IT! series for children living with diabetes
The first book in the series is, <u>The Little Red Sports Car</u>, ISBN: 978-0615132815
The second book in the series is, <u>Winston the Amazing Dog</u>, ISBN: 978-1478348498

All the books in the YOU CAN DO IT! series are available through Amazon.com and
Kindle, or email the author at: etroutt3@gmail.com

ISBN-13: 978-1484055571
ISBN-10: 1484055578

Printed in the United States of America

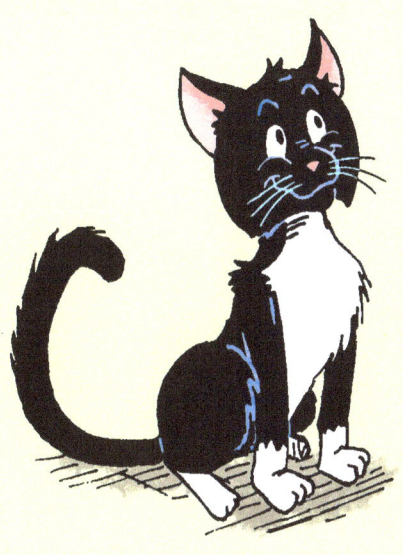

There once was a cat named Boots who was jet black and had little white booties on his feet and a little white dickey at his throat.

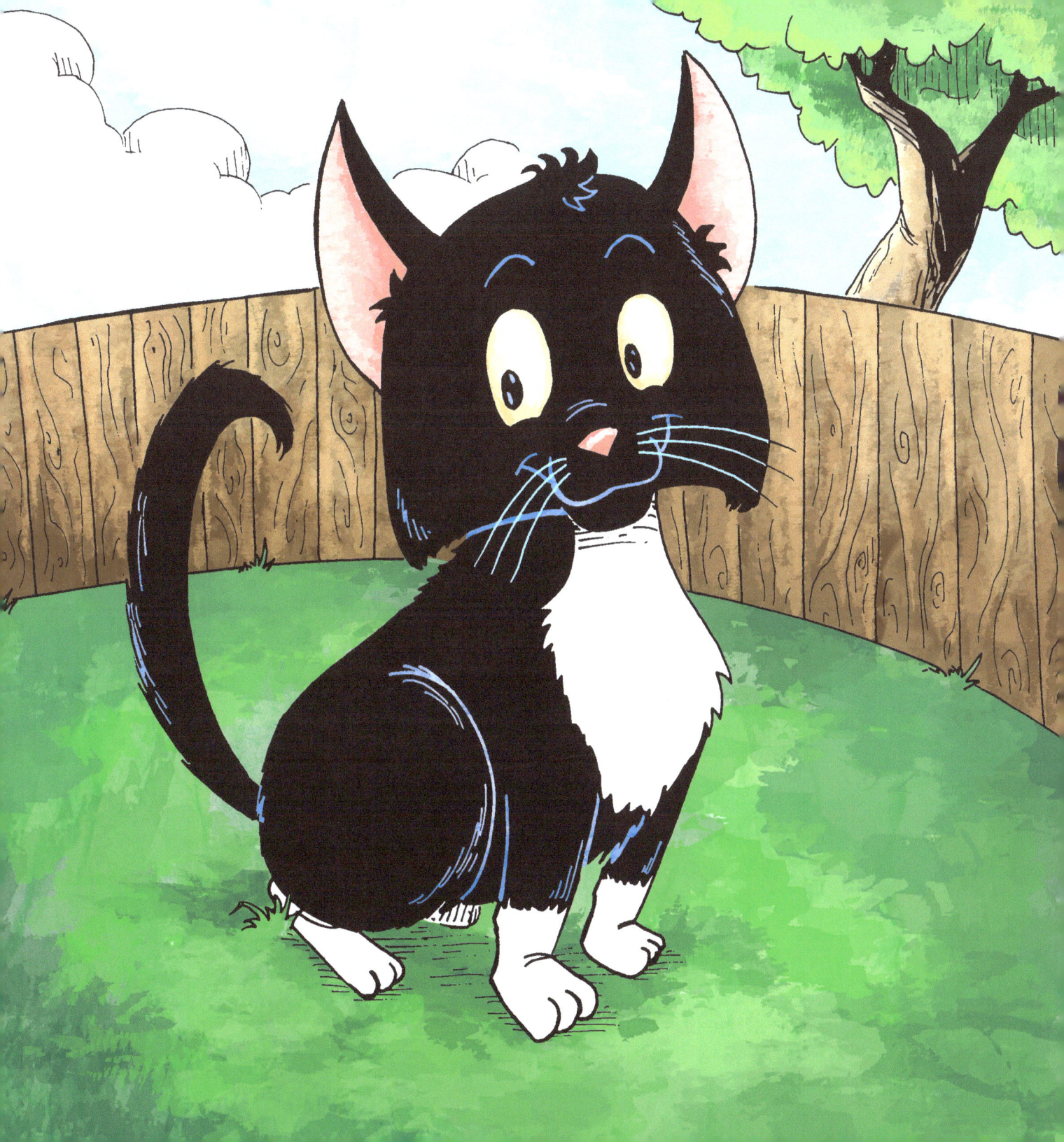

He was just a little kitten but he could do some marvelous things. For example, he used to watch how Ellie opened the door leading into the back yard and he figured out that the way to get outside was to turn the door knob. He tried! And he tried! Of course, he couldn't open the door as hard as he tried but he kept trying.

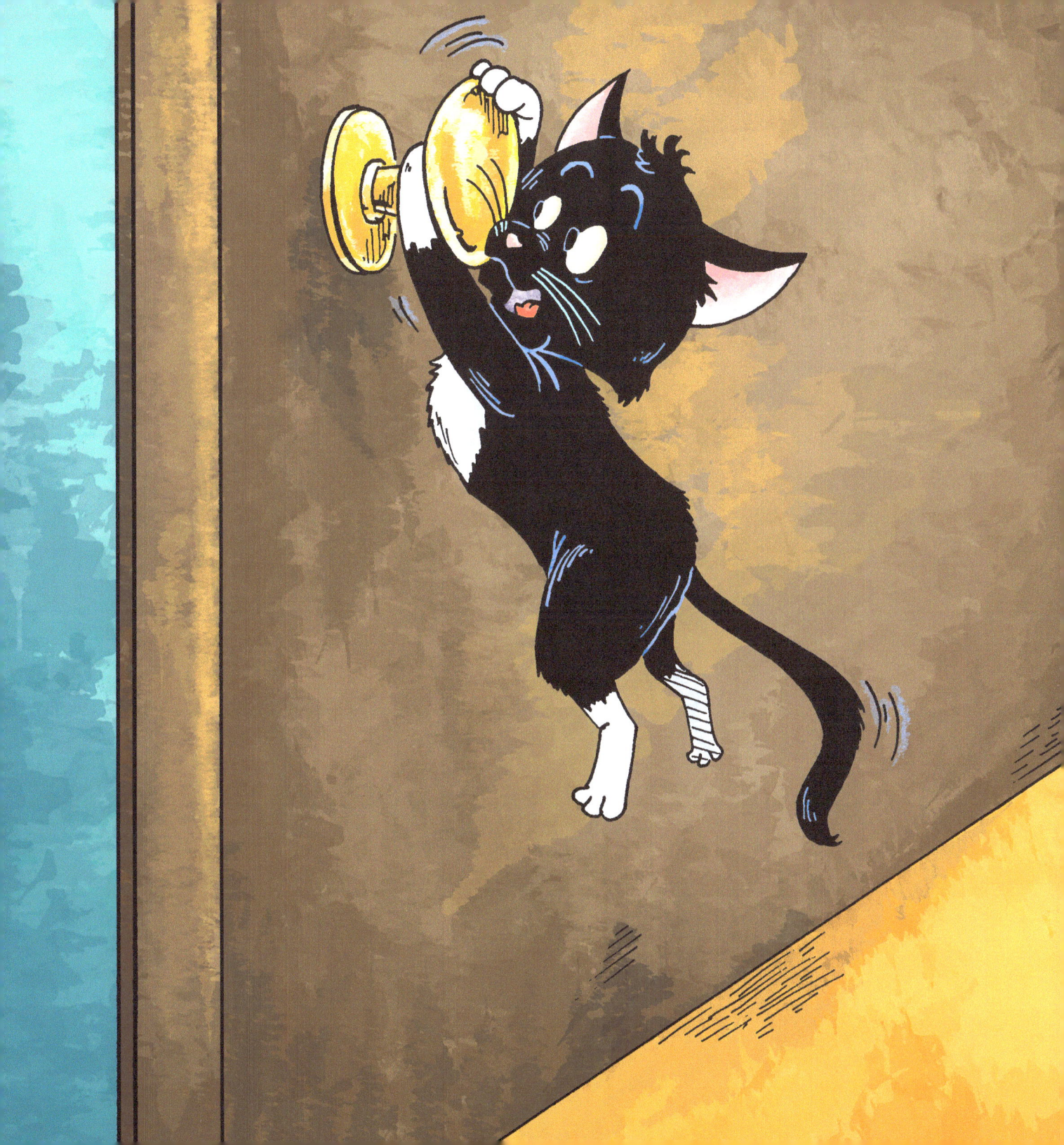

At Christmas time when Ellie put up a Christmas tree in the living room, the whole family enjoyed hanging the tinsel and the lights and the decorations. One year Ellie put a pretty little glass bell on one of the bottom branches. A little while later she was surprised to hear the soft tinkle of a bell and went to investigate. There was Boots, softly and carefully batting away at the bell!

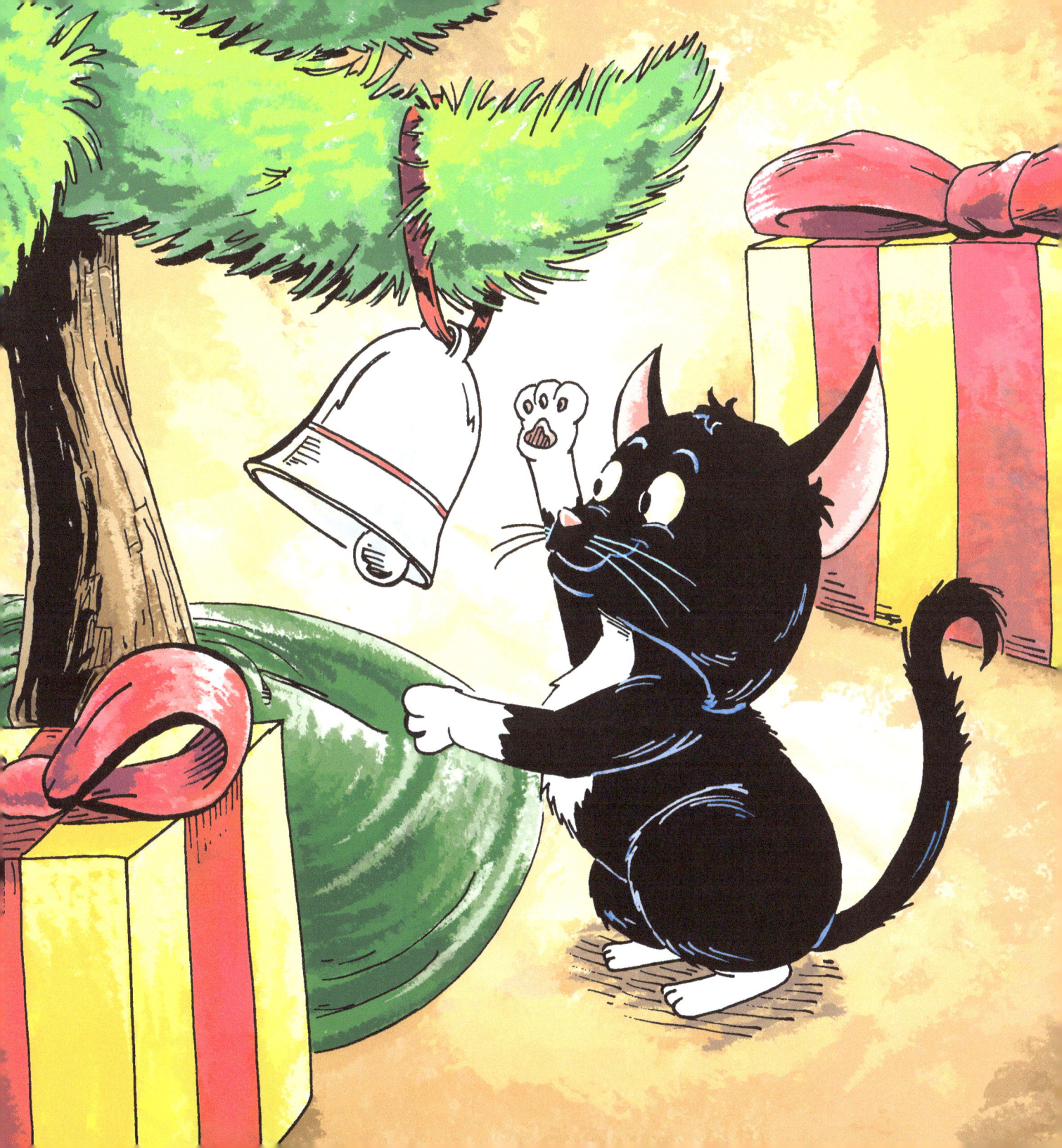

Boots didn't know he was just a little kitten. He believed he was the king of his own backyard.

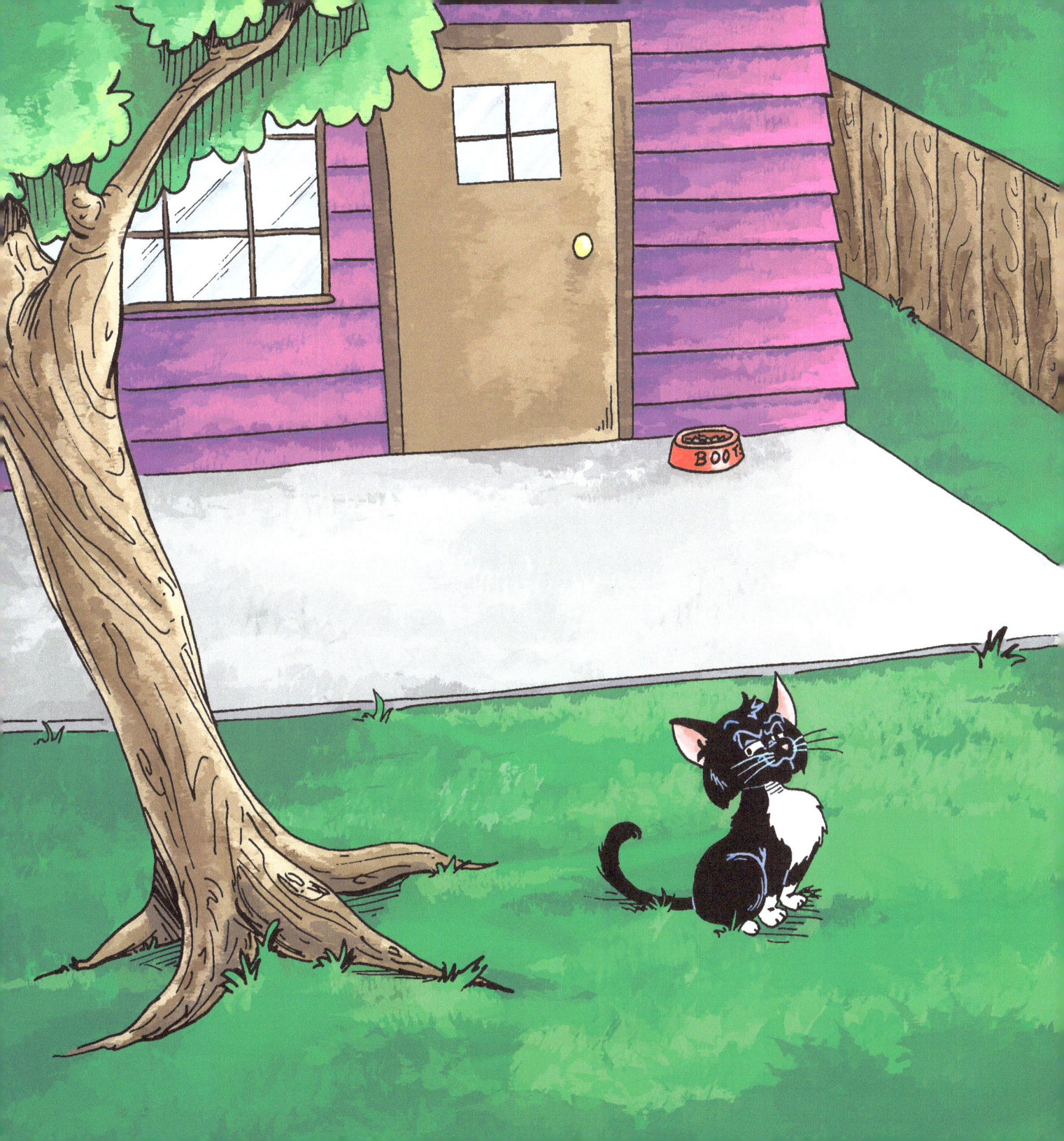

But he soon found out that he was badly mistaken because there was a big gray cat named Goliath who claimed the rights over Boot's backyard and every other backyard in the neighborhood.

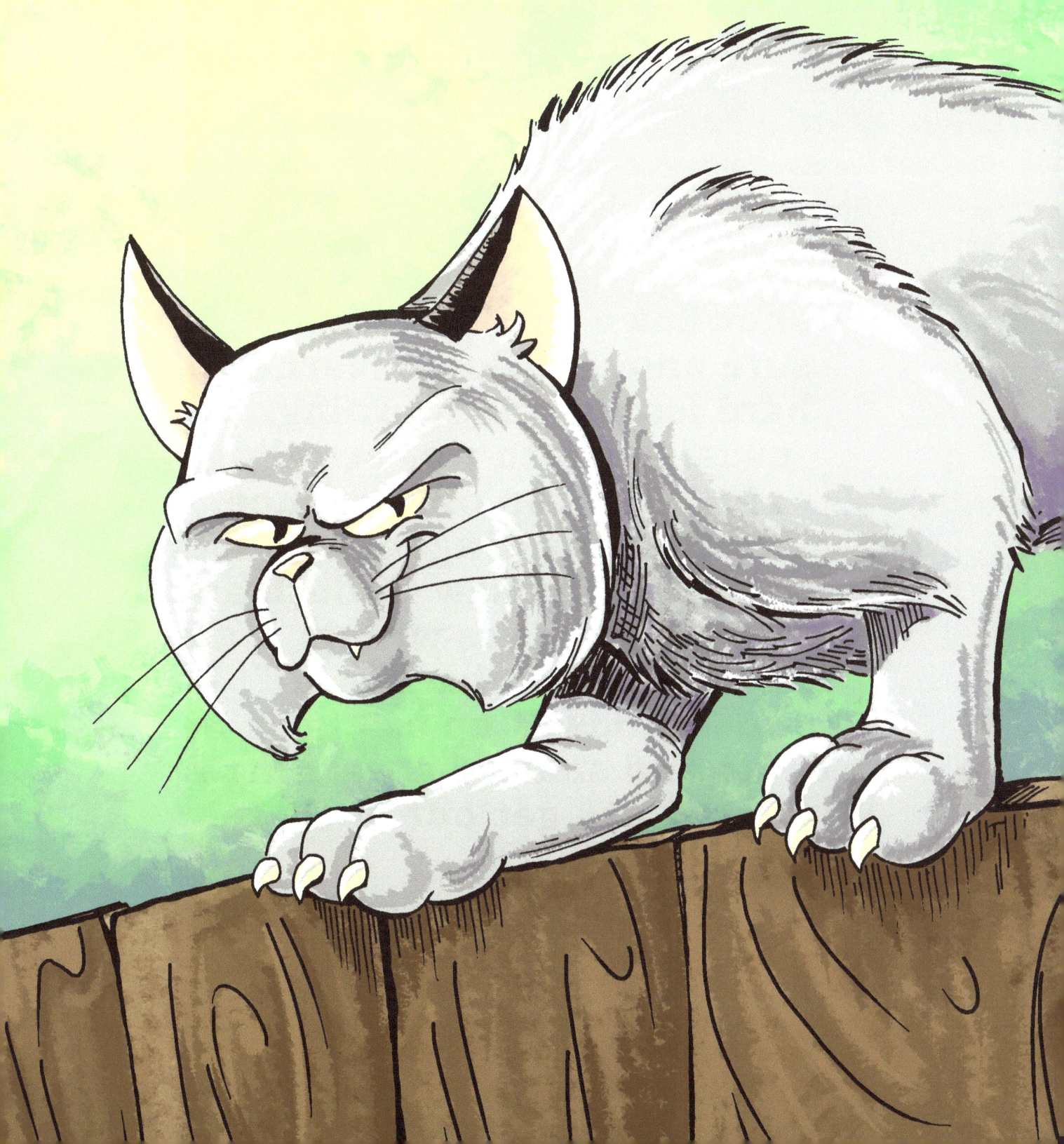

A showdown was inevitable! And sure enough, Boots learned a hard lesson one morning. As usual, Goliath was strolling along the top of the fence, patrolling his kingdom. Boots looked up and saw Goliath and thought, "This is wrong! I am king of my own backyard!" He puffed himself up as big as he could and snarled a warning to Goliath to get out of there.

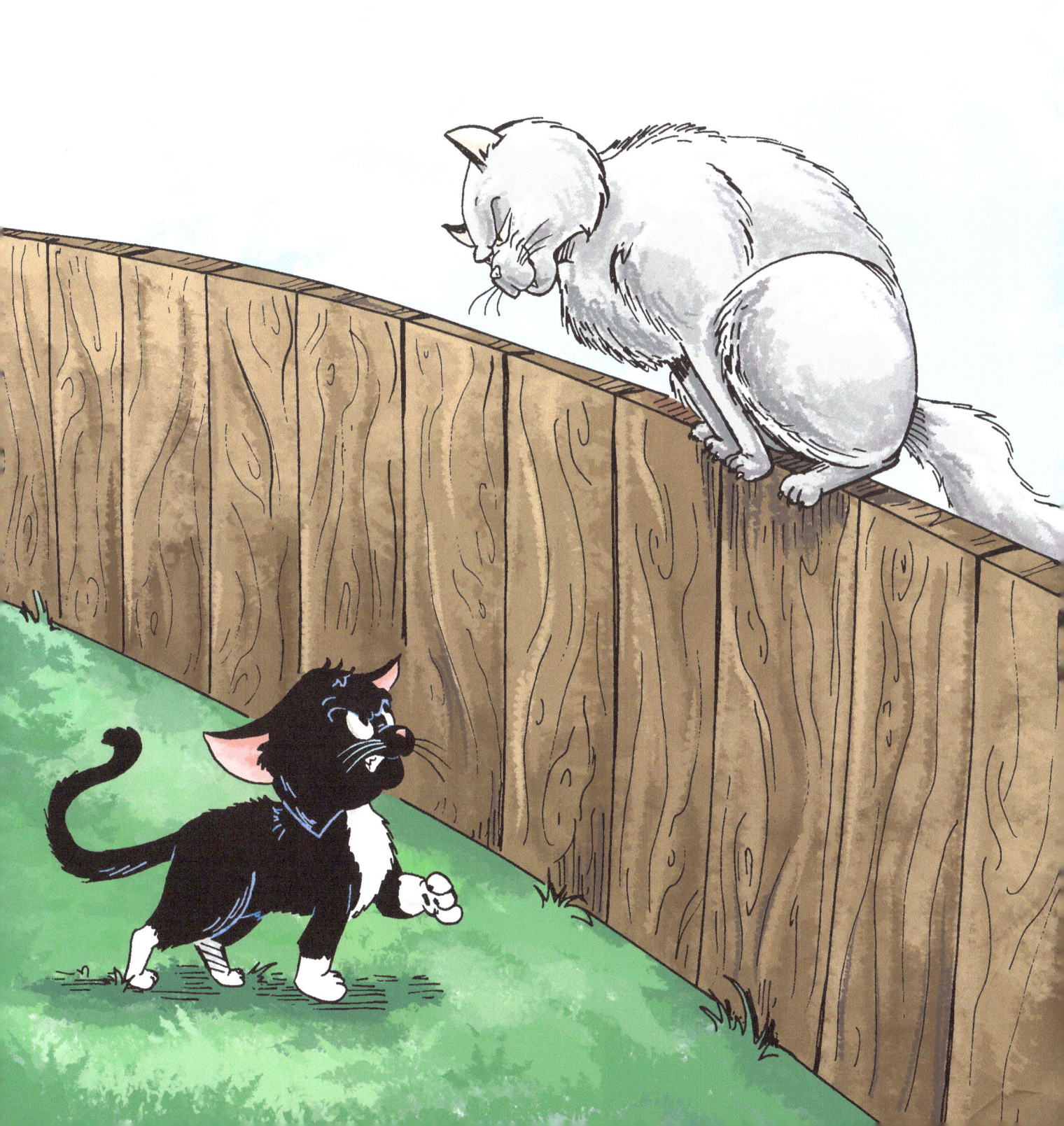

Goliath simply jumped down off the fence and gave this little upstart a thorough cuffing! Boots hardly knew what had hit him!

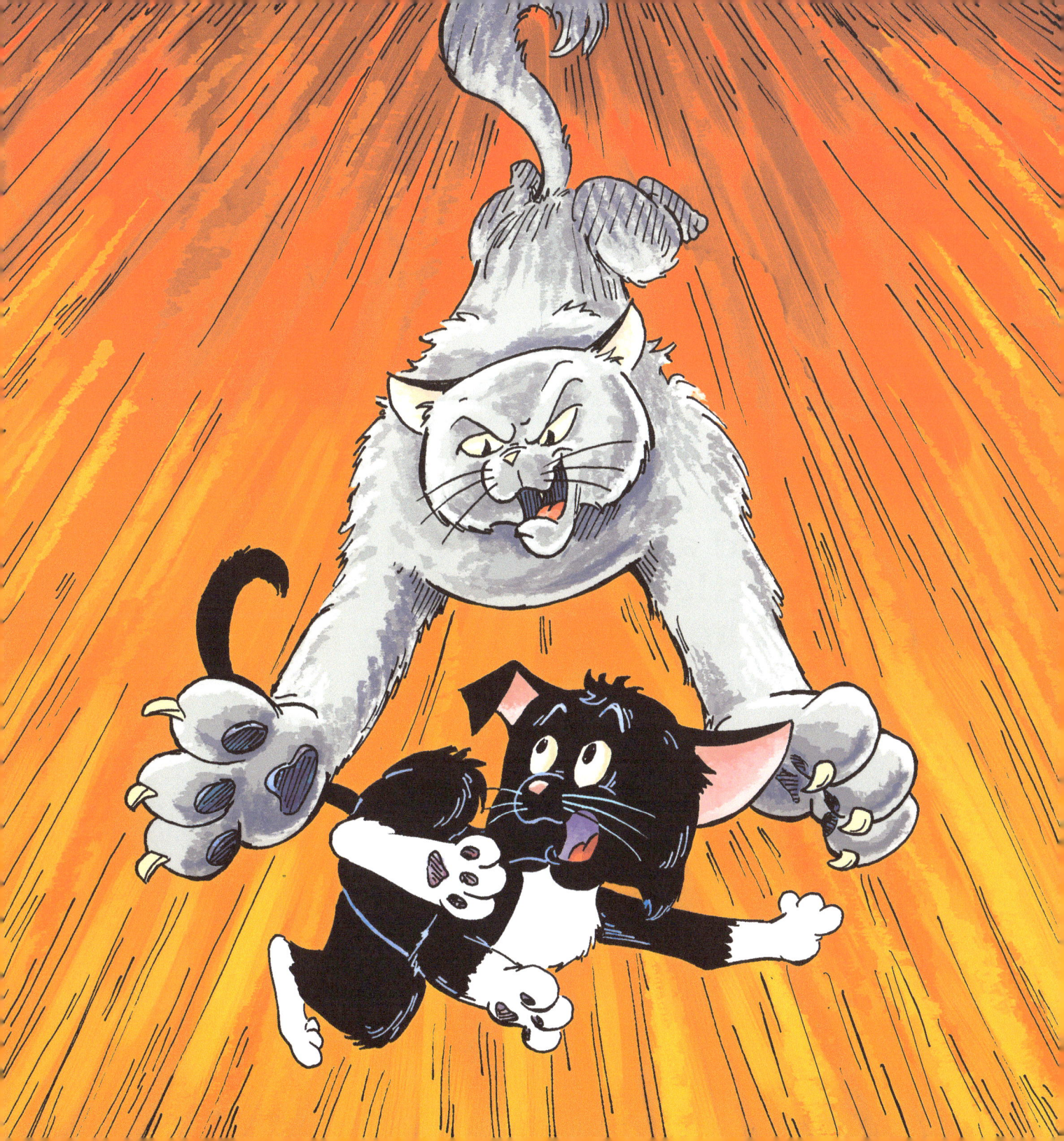

He limped to the back door and pitifully mewed to get in. Ellie dried up the blood as best she could and comforted him until his little heart stopped pounding and he was able to lap up some of the warm milk that she put down for him.

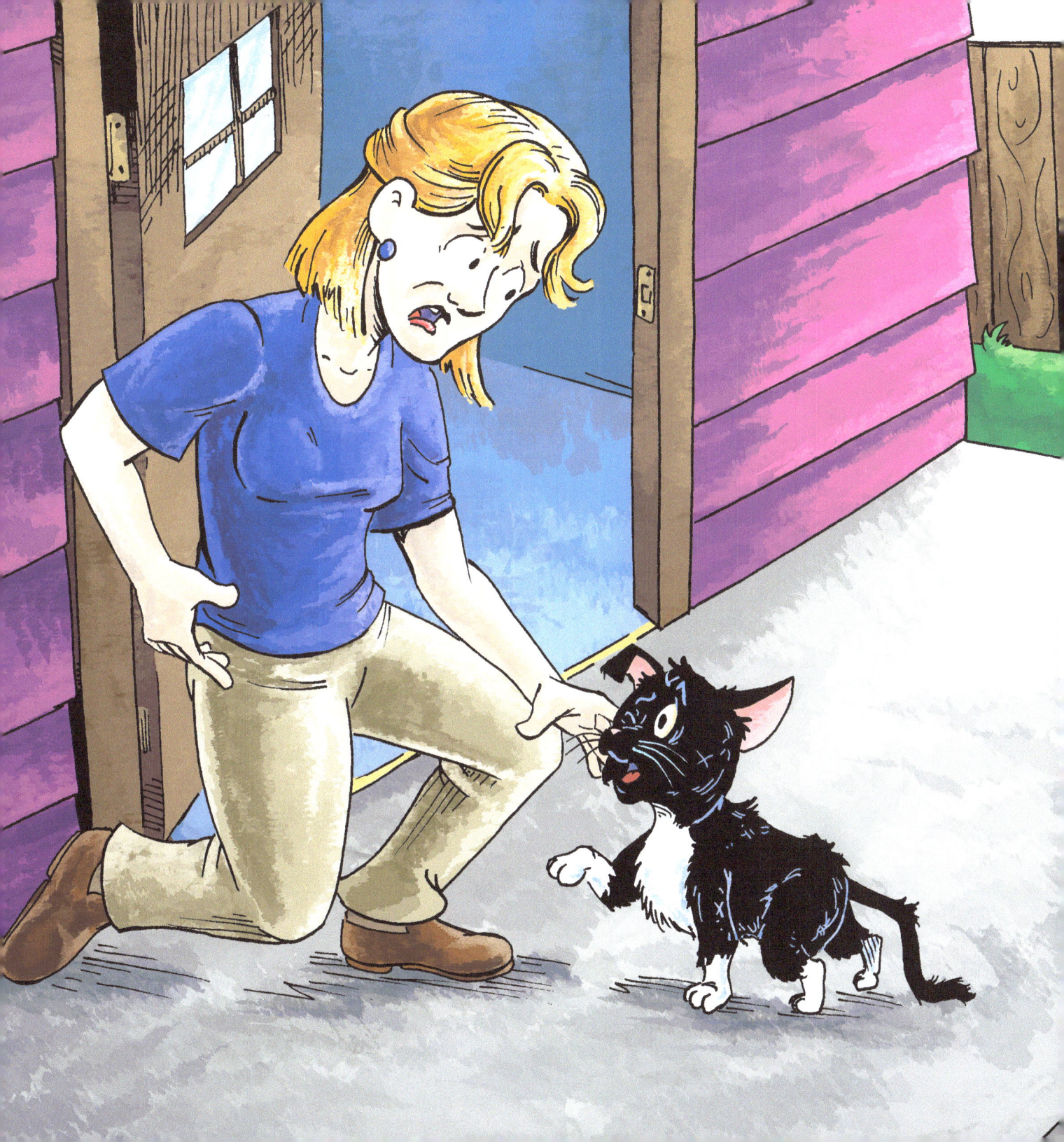

Goliath was clever and sneaky. Sometimes, he would wait until Boots was in another part of the back yard and then he would jump down off the fence and sneak over and steal the food that Ellie had put out for Boots. One day Boots caught him at this, but there was nothing he could do about it – he was too small.

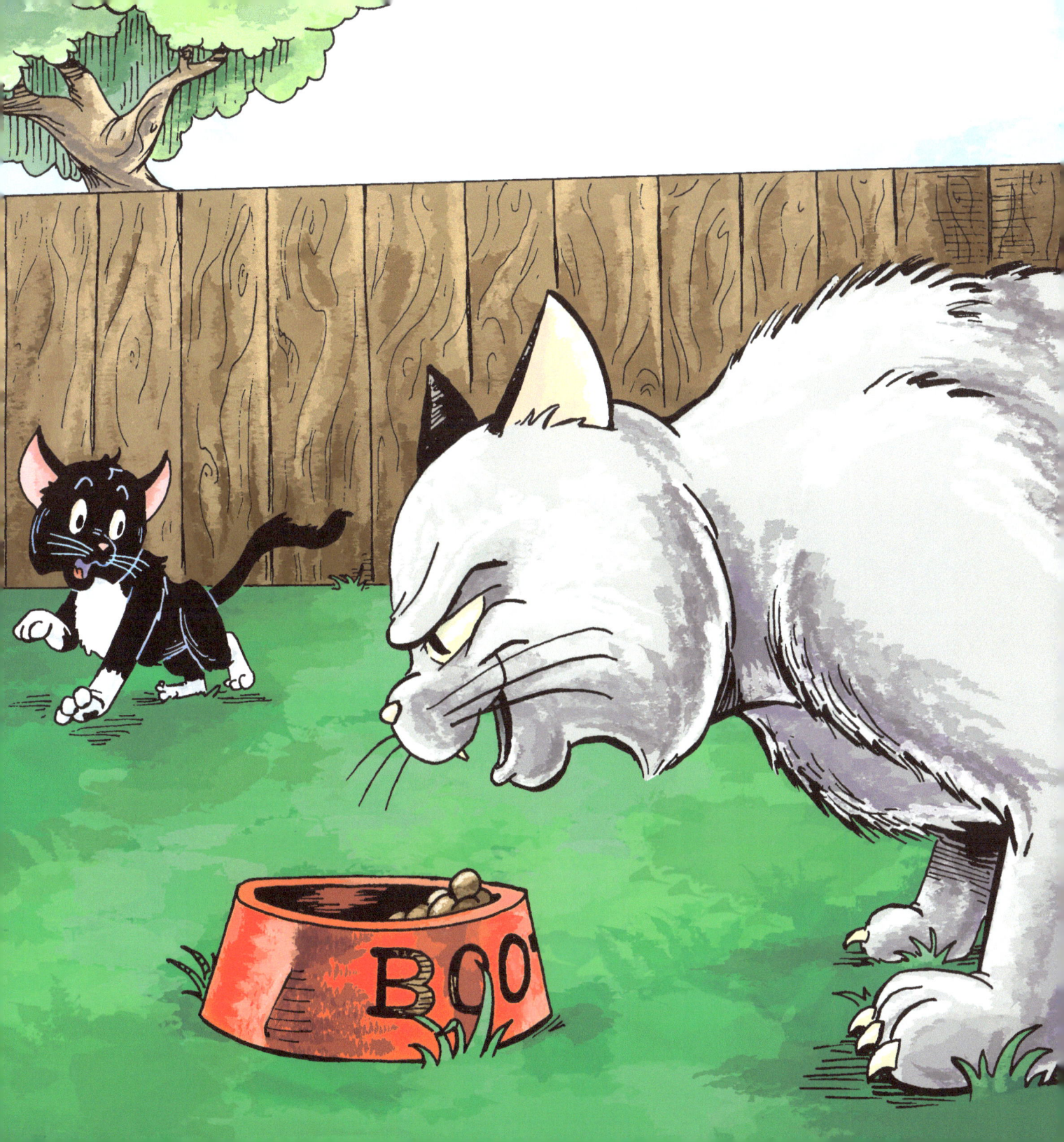

On another occasion, Goliath crept up on Boots and jumped on him from behind, scaring him half to death.

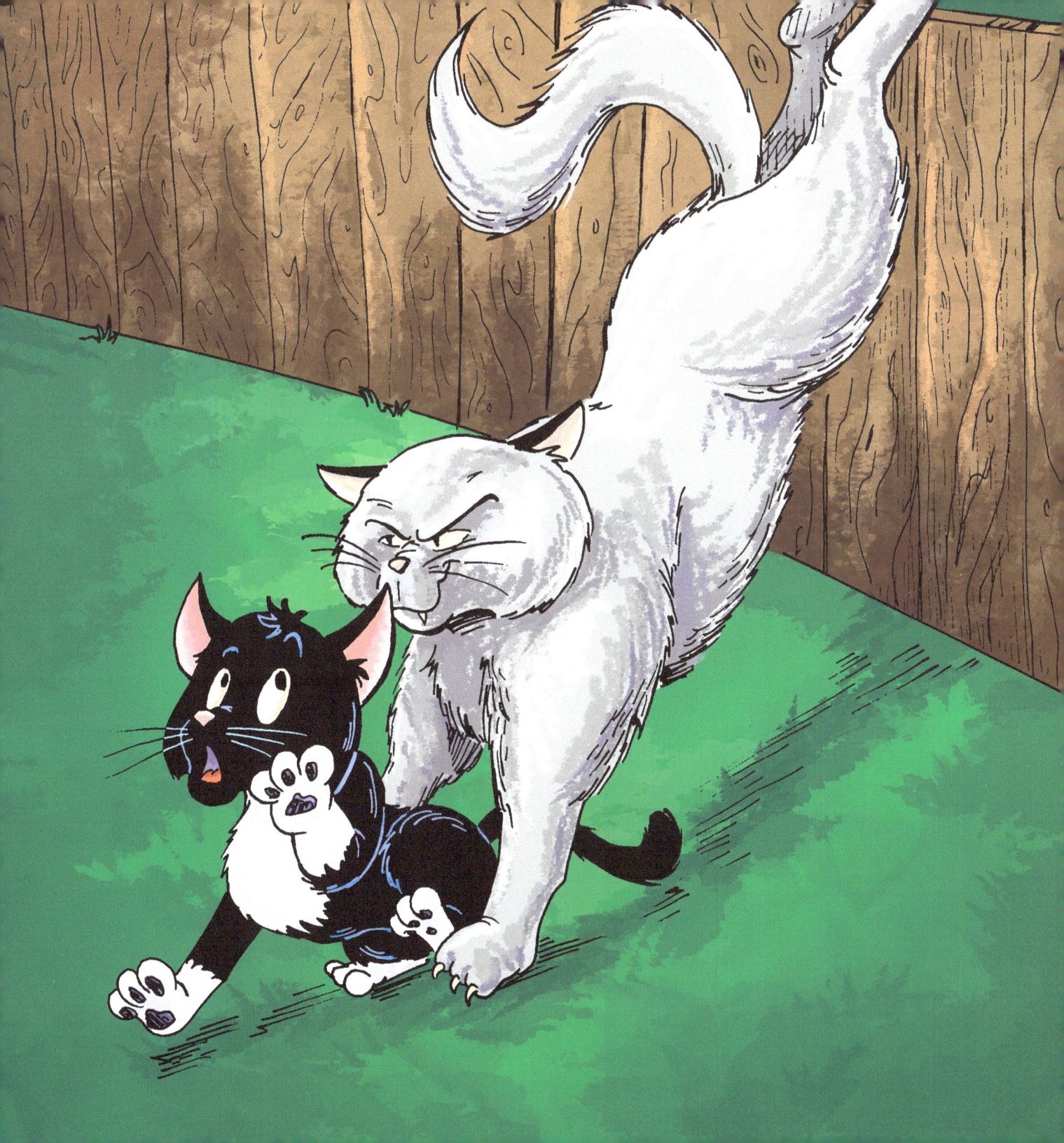

But Boots didn't stay a kitten
for long. Every day he got
bigger and smarter and stronger.

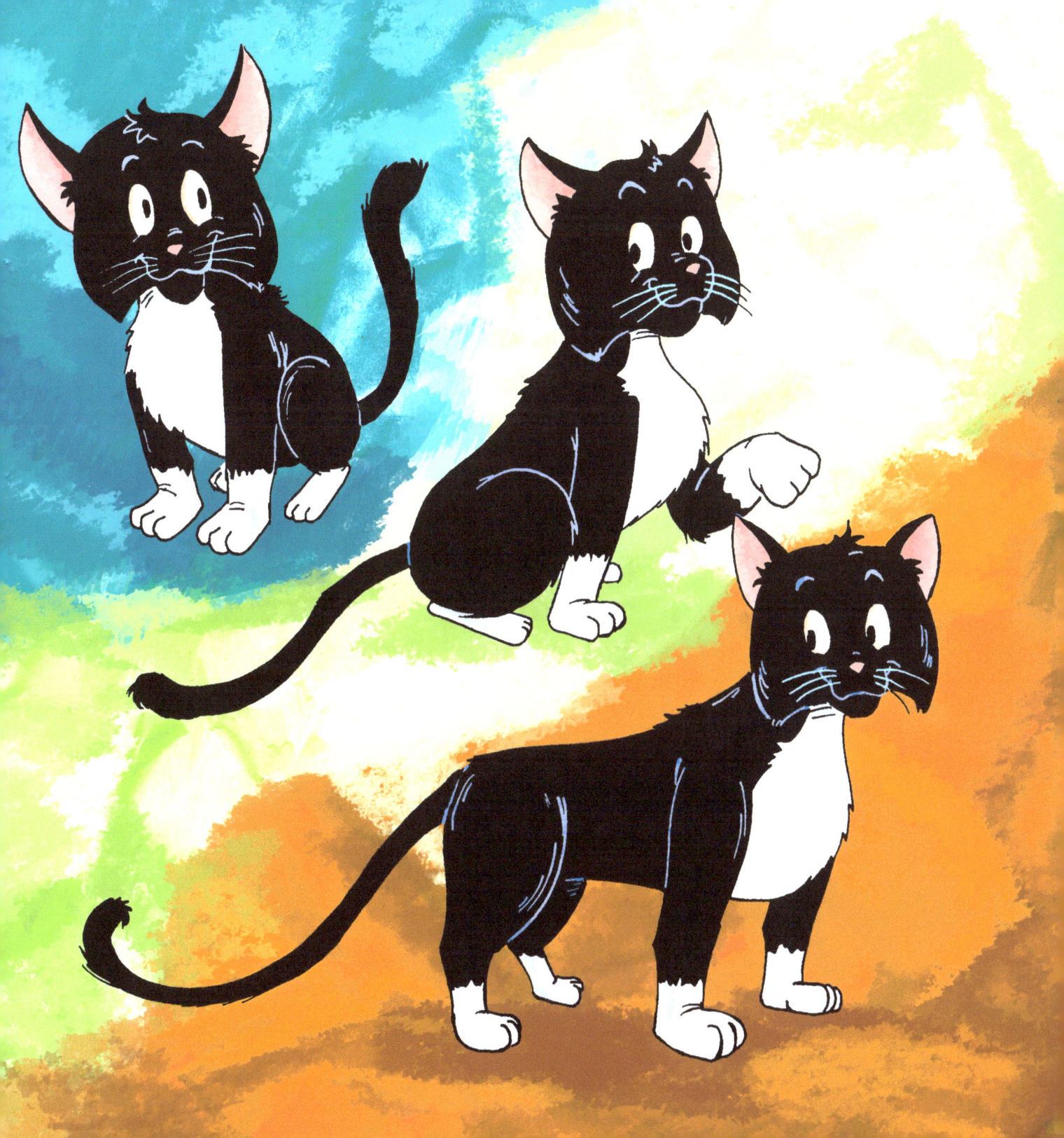

One day he was out in the back yard, and he spotted Goliath strolling along on the top of a neighbor's fence. At first, he was frightened and almost turned and ran back to the comfort of his own back door. But then he thought to himself, "Goliath has no right to be king of my back yard! I am the king!" So he stood his ground and looked defiantly up at this invader.

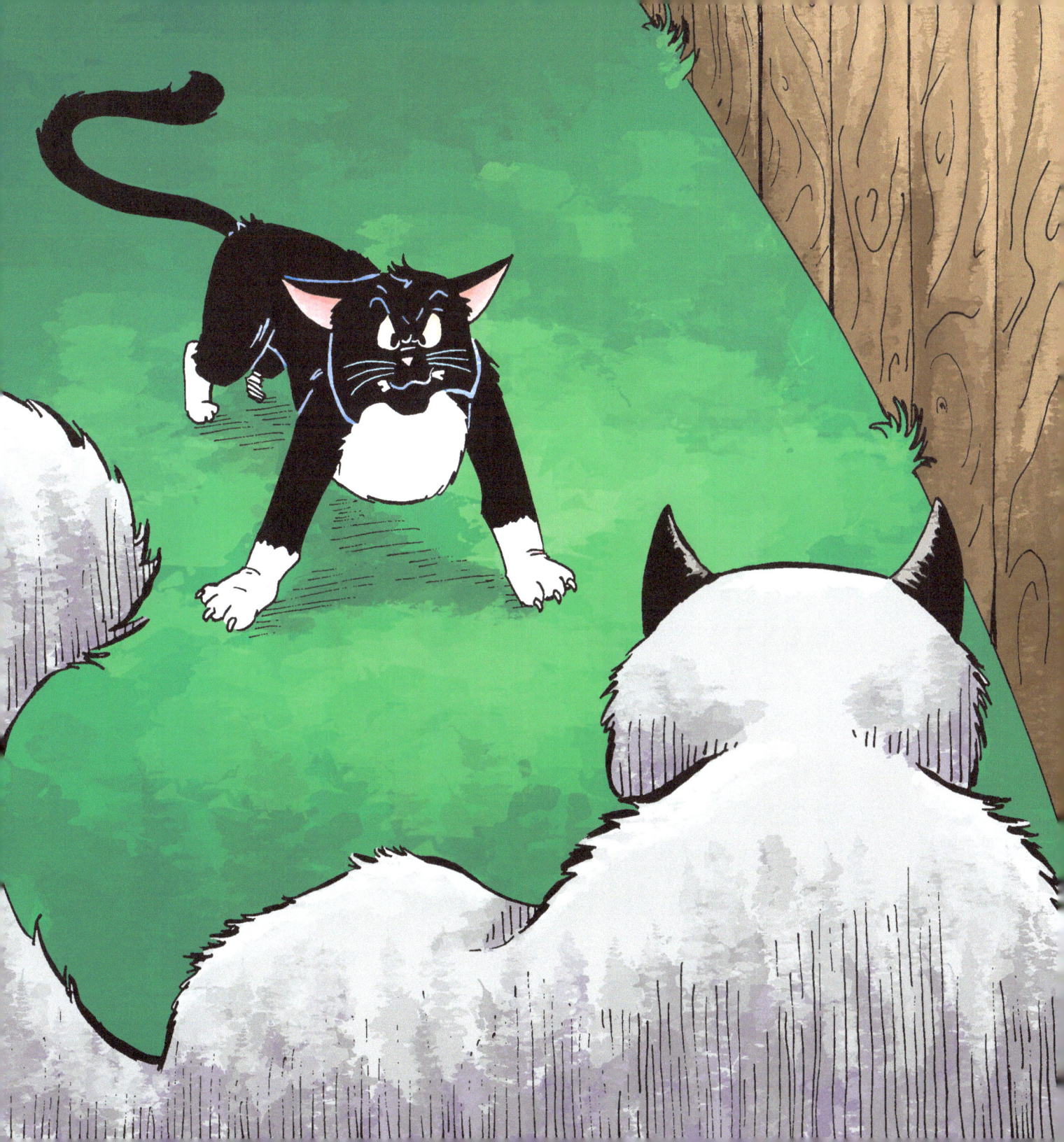

Goliath was a big cat and was used to making every other cat in the neighborhood shrink before him. So, he looked pityingly down at Boots and challenged him to do something about it. There was a lot of snarling and spitting as the two cats squared off for the duel of the century! But Boots was no longer a little kitten! He had sharpened his claws and put on weight and, although he wasn't as big as Goliath, he was confident that he could take back his own back yard!

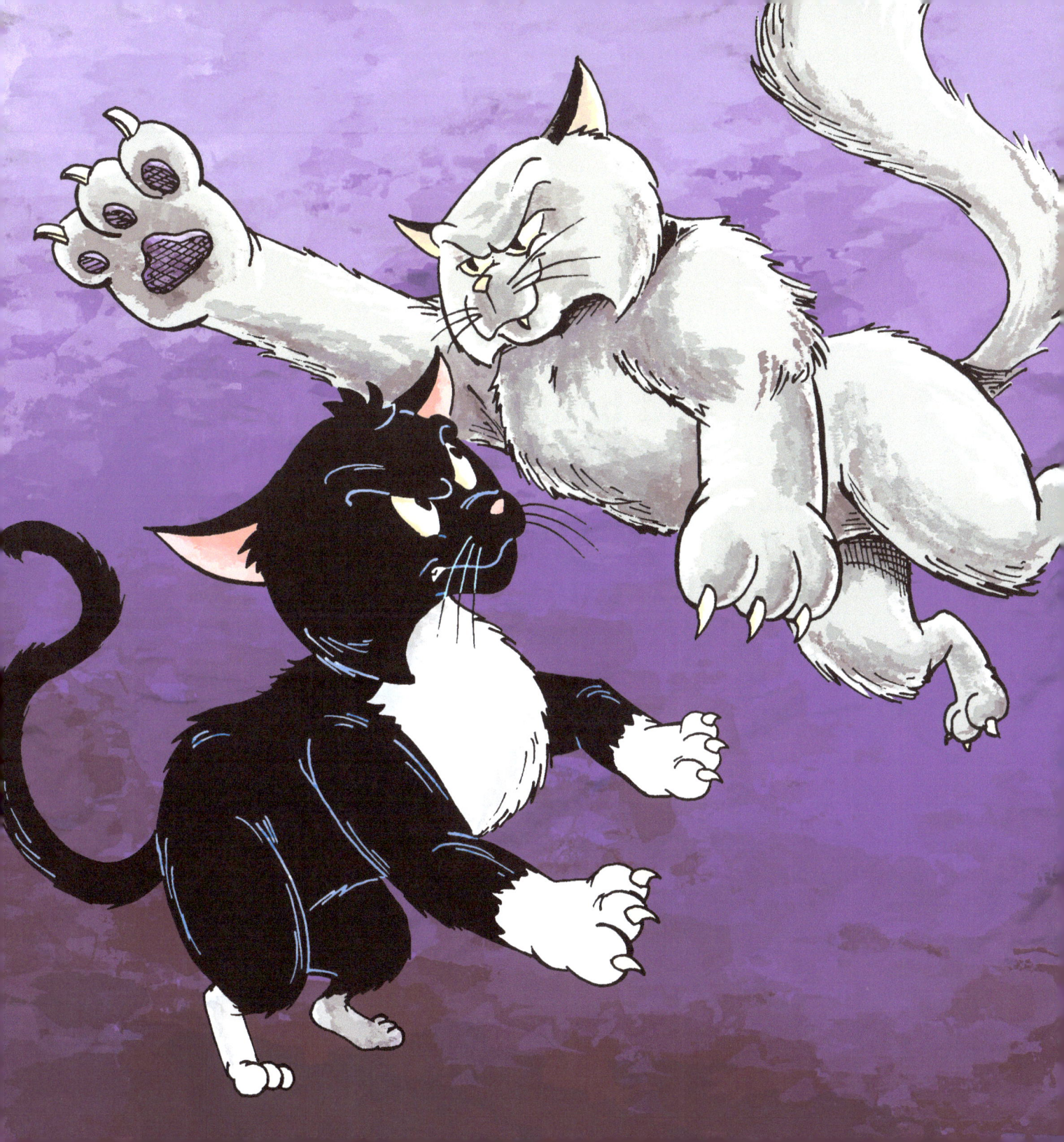

And that he did! The fight was short and brutal. And *this* time it was Goliath who limped home beaten and battered. He never challenged Boots again. And from that day on, Boots took pride in strolling around his domain without fear of a fight with Goliath or any other cat in the neighborhood.

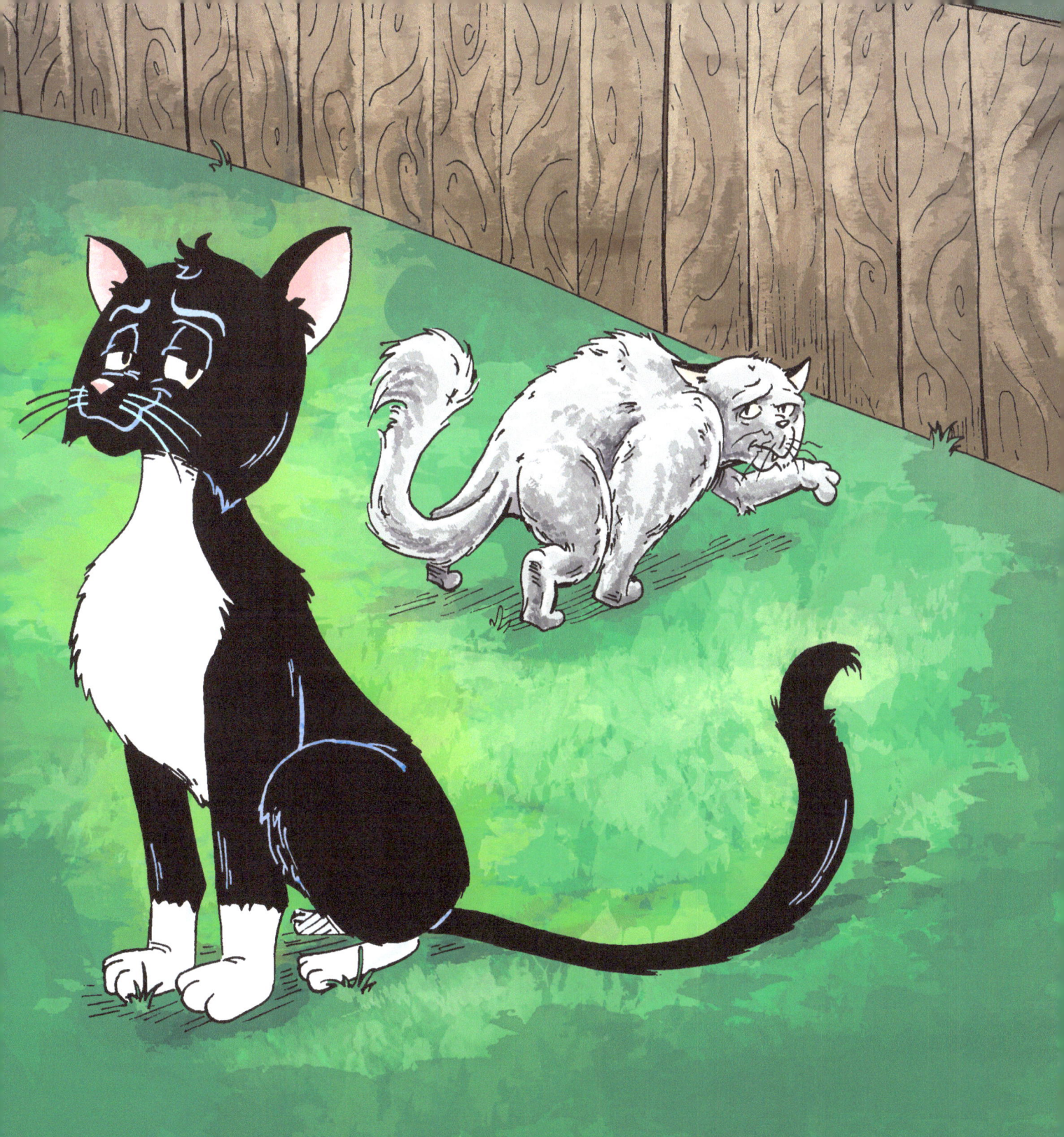

Ellie happened to have diabetes. And she saw that living with diabetes was, in many ways, like the contest for control that went on between Goliath and Boots, except that diabetes, for her, was an *on-going* battle. It was like always having to be on her guard against a wily opponent who was constantly trying to outsmart her. Sometimes diabetes won; sometimes she won.

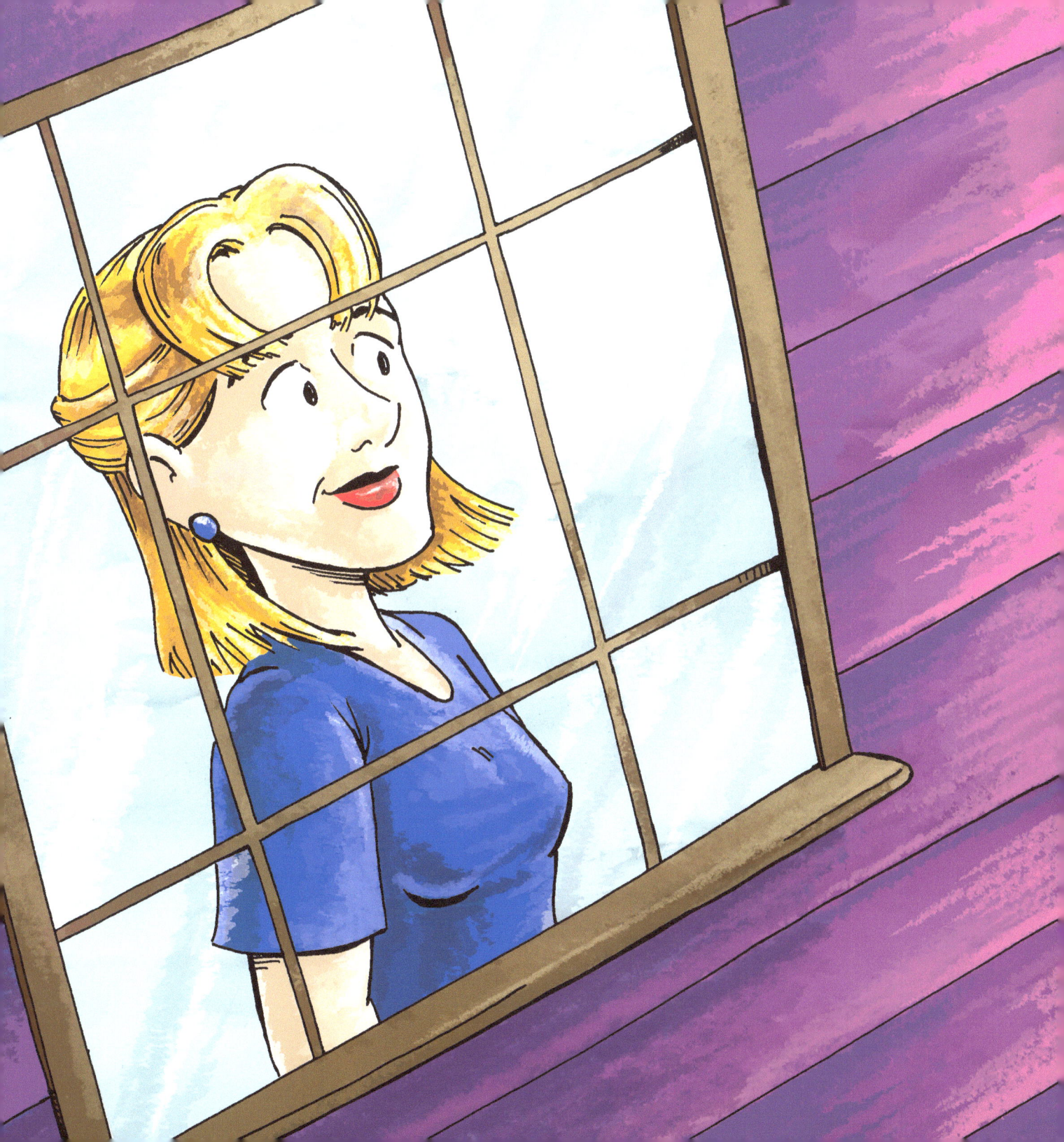

Ellie felt she could never let down her guard no matter how experienced she became in dealing with this clever, sneaky opponent.

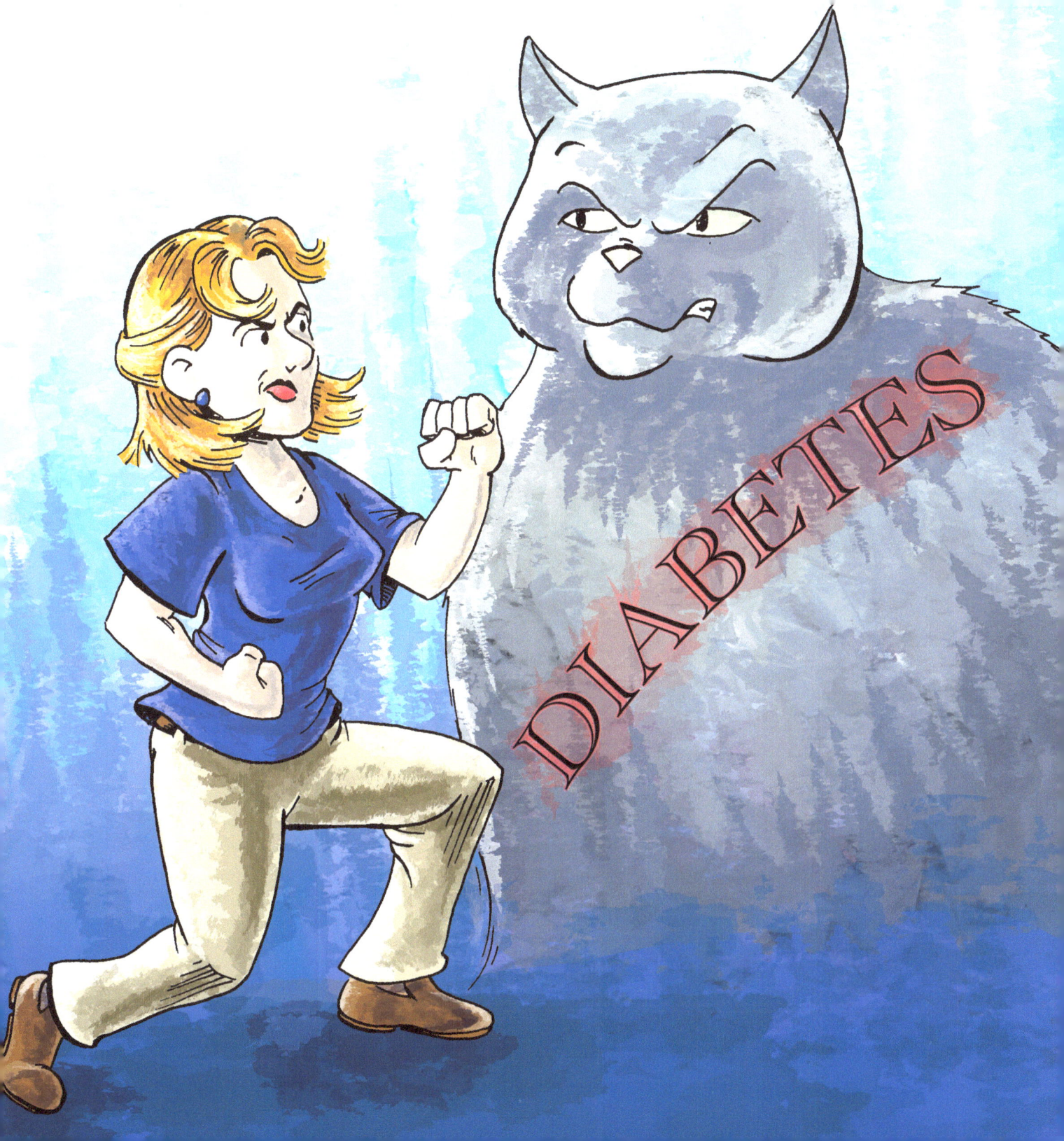

But the more she learned about diabetes and how it affected her, the more she felt able to defend herself against its tricks, and the more confident she became.

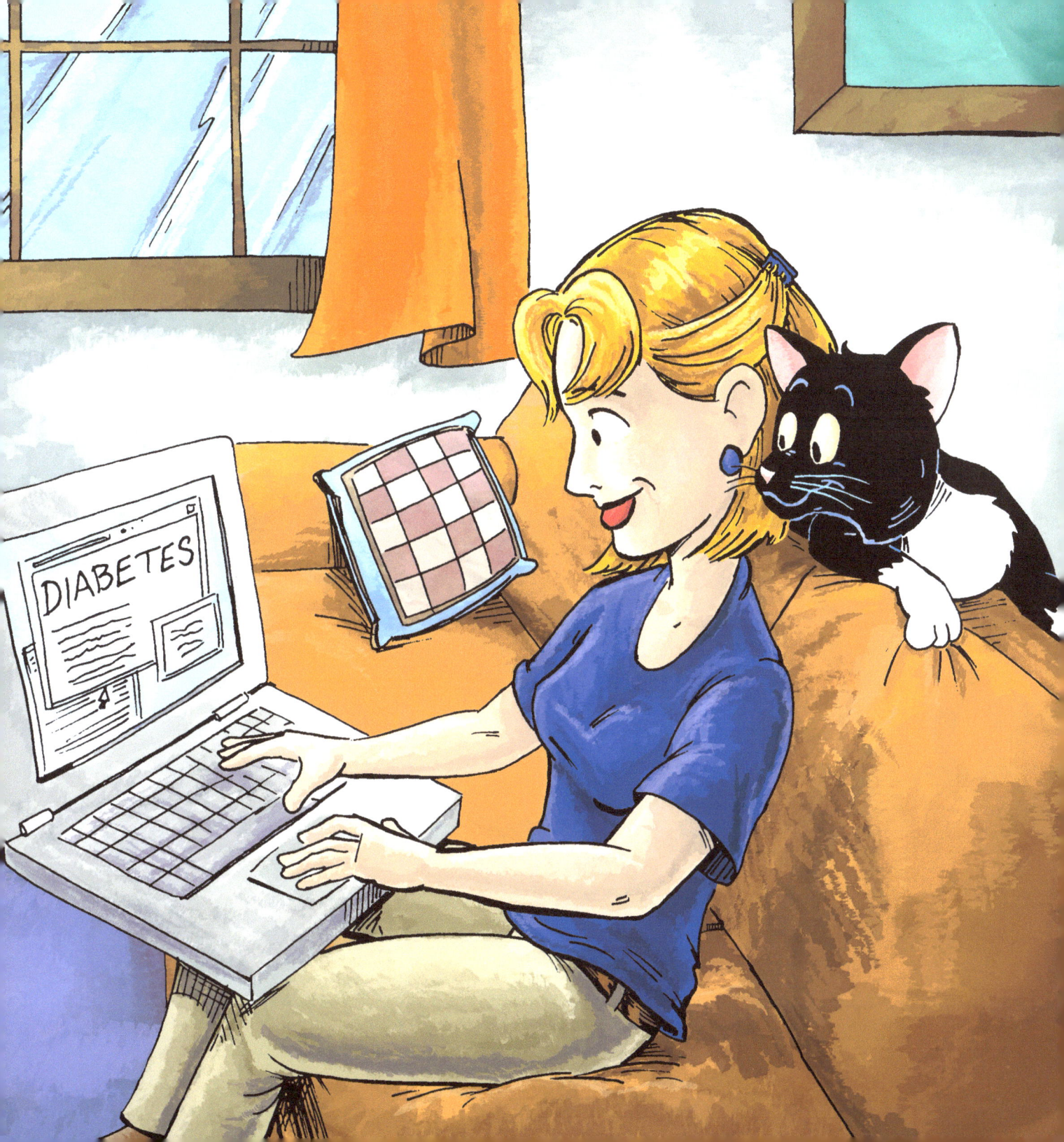

She was happy that she got lots of good help from skilled medical people who had a basic, solid understanding of this disease and could help her fight her daily battle.

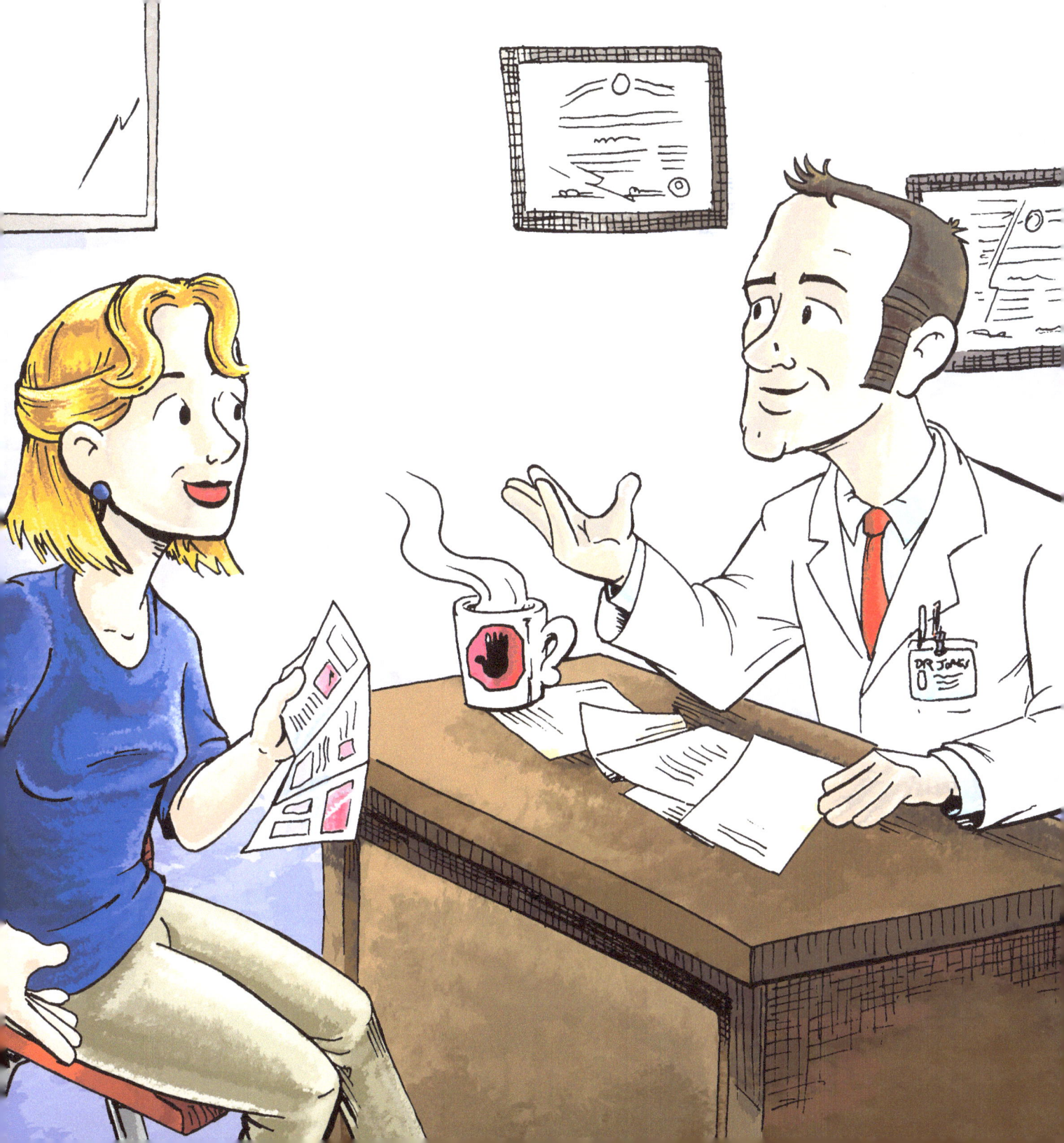

But Ellie knew that no matter how much help she got from them, nobody could fight this battle for her. Like Boots, she had to fight the battle for herself. And win!

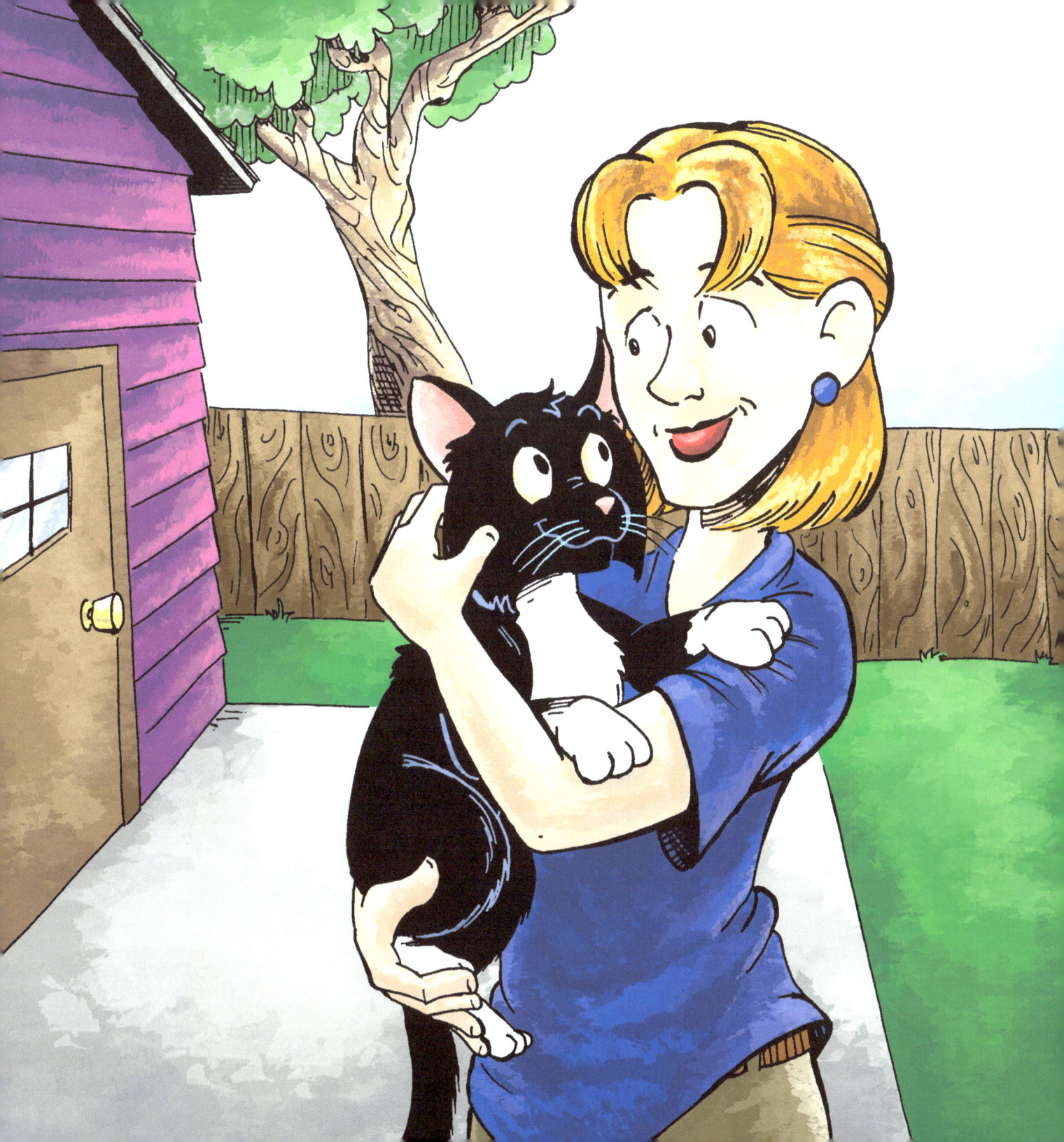

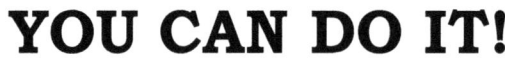

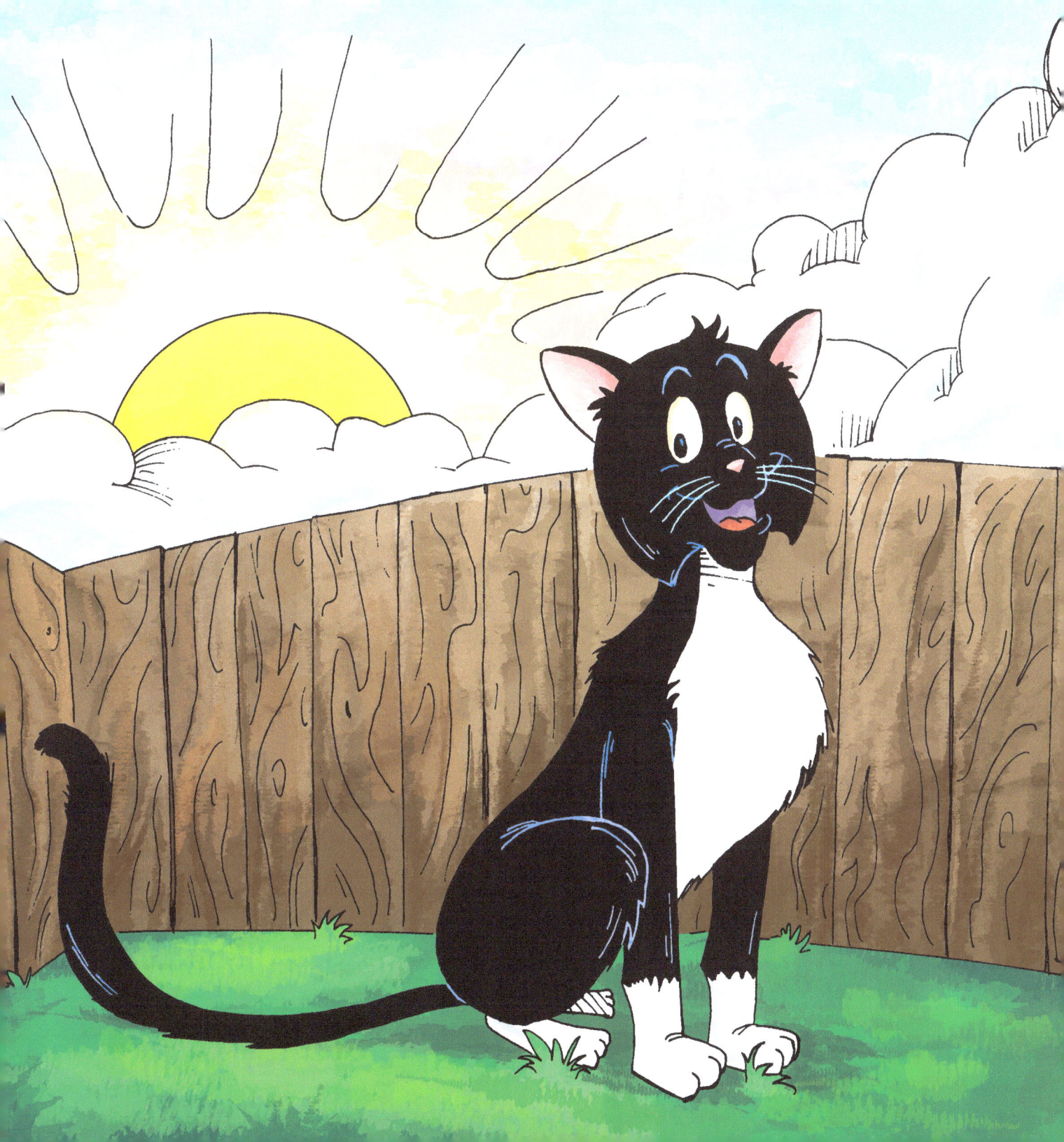

www.ingramcontent.com/pod-product-compliance
Lightning Source LLC
Chambersburg PA
CBHW041522280526
45792CB00004B/1341